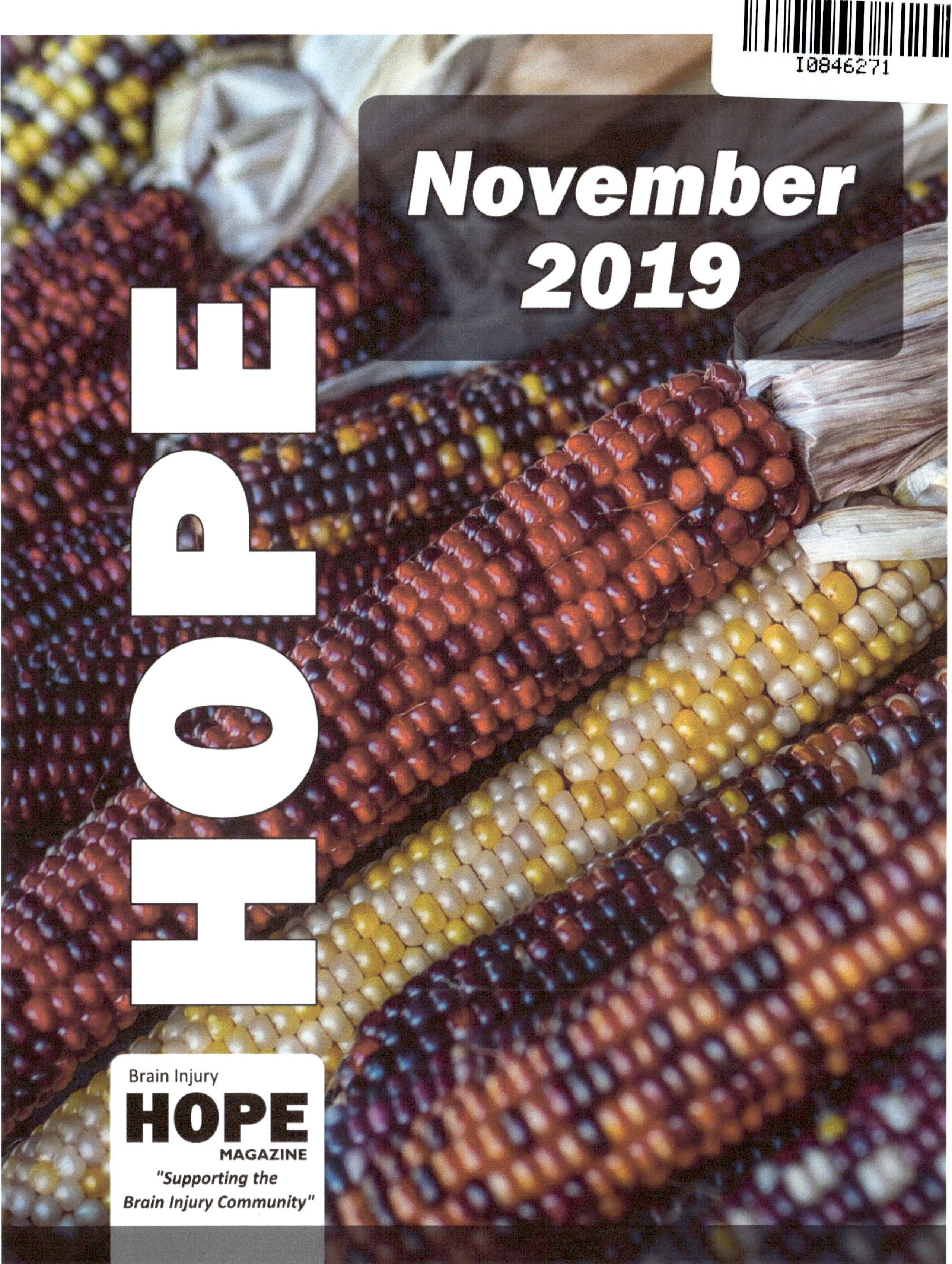

November
2019
HOPE
Brain Injury
HOPE
MAGAZINE
"Supporting the
Brain Injury Community"
I0846271

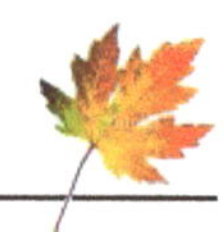

HOPE MAGAZINE

Serving the Brain Injury Community Since 2015

November 2019

Publisher
David A. Grant

Editor
Sarah Grant

Our Contributors

Sandra Bastinelli
Patrick Brigham
Debra Gorman
Susan Hayes
JoAnne Silver Jones
Tracie Massie
Donna O'Donnell Figurski
Isaac Peterson

Welcome to the November 2019 Issue of HOPE Magazine!

In the four-and-a-half years since we launched HOPE Magazine, we've featured contributing writers from around the world. Brain injury knows no geographic bounds. Both acquired as well as traumatic brain injury can happen to anyone, anywhere.

Life is indeed so much more fragile than most of us ever give thought to.

This month we are excited to bring you several first-time contributors. Their stories are real, raw, and authentic. It takes a great deal of courage to open up and share what is perhaps the most difficult chapter of one's life, yet it is in that courageous sharing that healing comes to pass.

Join me in welcoming Susan, Joanne, Sandra and Isaac to our family of contributors. I'd love to hear your feedback about this month's issue. Feel free to reach out to me directly at david@tbihopeandinspiration.com.

Peace to all,

David A. Grant
Publisher

Contents

THINK ABOUT THIS

Every day, almost 200 people in the United States die from a TBI.
-CDC Statistic

QUOTABLE

"I have always had a bad memory, as far back as I can remember."
-Lewis Thomas

DID YOU KNOW

This month's issue of HOPE Magazine is our 58th consecutive issue!

A SCUBA Ballet

By Debra Gorman

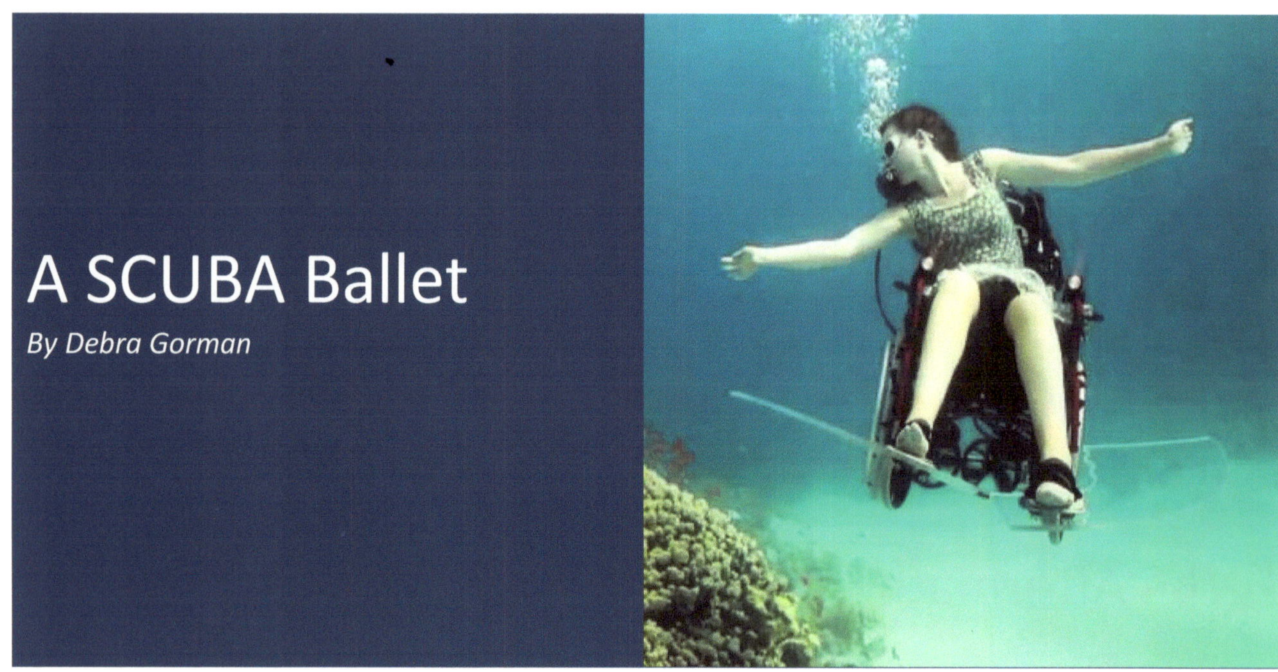

I just watched a video of a woman's scuba dive in a wheelchair. It's on YouTube and I don't remember her name, but that doesn't seem very important at the moment. What I remember most clearly is her message that her perspective from a wheelchair is unique and beautiful. In the video she wore a dress that lifted and flowed around her in graceful patterns, as did her long dark hair. She was strapped in and used her arms to twirl as she rose or descended in the deep water, like a solo scuba ballet.

It got me thinking how I often let my brain injury disable me, tell me that my worth is less than when I was able-bodied, strong and youthful. When I start reflecting more about the lessons I can learn and benefit from, and less about my perceived losses, I will more fully appreciate how blessed I am.

It's now nearly 2020. I wrote the above two paragraphs on May 30, 2015. It was probably meant to be the beginning of a blog post, but I stopped there and filed it away, not knowing where to go with it. What strikes me first in rereading this is how little I seem to have grown as a person over the last five years. I would have expected that by now I would be more accepting of my current life. I expected to be wiser and more mature.

I'll give myself a little credit. A year ago, I would have been more frustrated with

> **"One thing I'm learning is to give myself grace, forgiveness and compassion."**

myself at not being further along the path toward enlightenment. One thing I'm learning is to give myself grace, forgiveness and compassion. I don't currently believe I'll ever stop grieving over my new, unrequested, uncomfortable life, but that's okay. I will always try to make the best of it. It is advantageous that I recognize grief for what it is and "go with the flow." Because of the way my life is playing out, I'm learning things about people and life in general that would not have been accessible to me before. As a result, I am more capable of loving and giving in a meaningful way.

I looked online for information about the underwater performer. Her name is Susan Felicity Austin. She is a disabled British artist. Her videos are freely available to watch on YouTube. I also watched two Ted Talks where she spoke and showed a video of her dive. In both talks Susan said something I can't easily wrap my head around. She said she experienced tremendous freedom when she got her new electric wheelchair. Freedom? In a wheelchair?

After watching one of Susan's Ted Talks again, I heard her say she had been in a wheelchair for sixteen years before getting the powered chair. I didn't catch it the first time and that's significant. I can now understand why a powered chair would feel liberating.

I'll never forget my UN-liberating use of a wheelchair. It was four months after my brain hemorrhage. My husband and I were trying to shop for Christmas. I felt the shopping trip was a disaster. I thought that by using the chair I would maximize our time and fight fatigue. Otherwise, I knew I would have been unable to continue after thirty to forty-five minutes. I found it frustrating to be so out of control. Stores were crowded and noisy and I couldn't reach the things that I wanted to take a closer look at. I couldn't communicate loud enough to stop, turn or slow down. John would have been happy to do whatever I asked but wasn't very good at reading my mind. We didn't accomplish much that day, and I vowed to never use the wheelchair again. So far, knock on wood, I haven't had to.

If I were not on this planet right now, living through all I do, I would not have enjoyed the last several wondrous weeks. I have two beautiful new granddaughters, the second granddaughter was born on our fourteenth wedding anniversary, We recently flew out west where I witnessed the love and wedding of a young family member.

"If I were not on this planet right now, living through all I do, I would not have enjoyed the last several wondrous weeks."

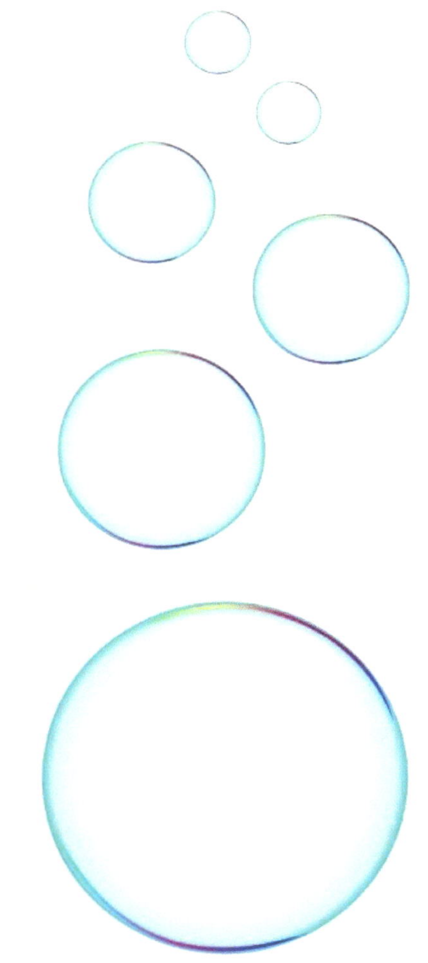

I enjoyed special meals and conversations with delightful extended family, some of whom live on the other end of the country and we had never met. I was completely charmed by the warmth extended to me by my husband's family.

The biggest lesson that I learn from all of this is to simply pay attention, to pay attention to wonder and beauty in its various forms and practice gratitude. Gratitude makes all the difference. Everything that happens has a purpose to benefit us. It's our job to look carefully and respond appropriately. Life isn't always difficult and painful, but it frequently is. Sometimes we get to experience the promise of a new life and know great love. Other times, we need to dig down deep to extract meaning from life events that will provide strength to continue. That's okay too. Ultimately, life is what we decide it will be. As long as we can think, we have the power to choose, and today I choose to live the best life possible.

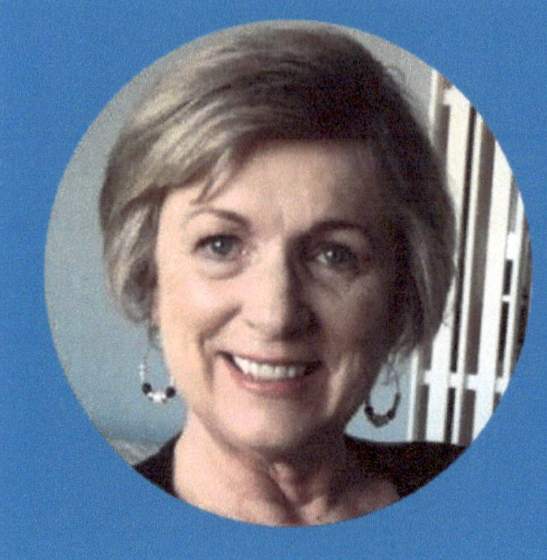

Meet Debra Gorman

Debra Gorman was fifty-six years old in 2011 when she experienced a cavernous angioma on her brain stem, causing her brain to bleed. Four months later she sustained a subdural hematoma. She later learned that she also had suffered a stroke during one of those events. She finds a creative outlet in writing. She enjoys writing for her children and grandchildren and has written articles that have been published for hospice, local newspapers, and Hope magazine. Currently, she writes for her blog, entitled Graceful Journey at debralynn48.wordpress.com.

Let's Get Social!

What do over 30,000 people from 26 countries and five continents all have in common? They are all members of our vibrant Facebook family at /TBIHopeandInspiration

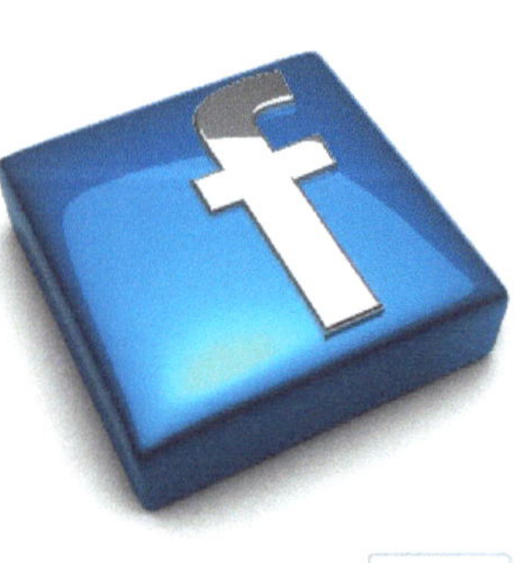

Join our Facebook Family Today!

The Aftermath

By Tracie Massie

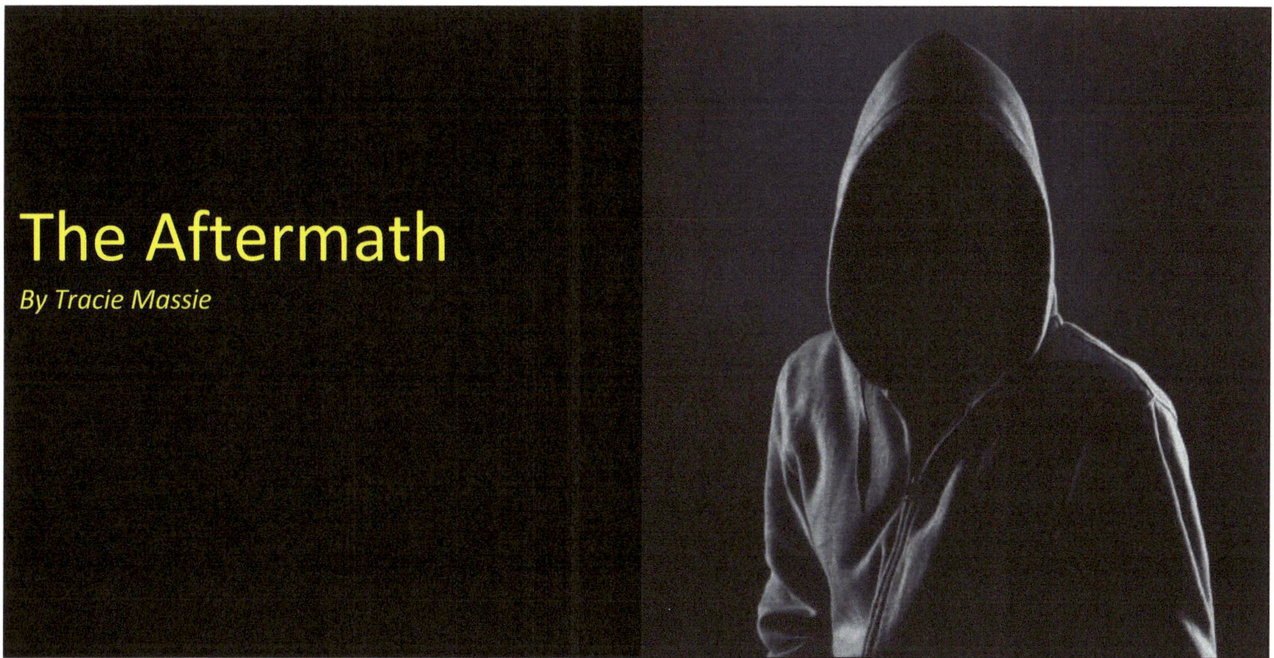

It's been thirteen years. Some days it seems longer, and on other days it seems like just yesterday. I have a picture of my son that was taken a few weeks before his car accident. It is my favorite picture of him. This picture shows everything that he was before the accident.

My son was quiet, gentle, kind and generous. I'm not saying that is all gone, but since his accident and subsequent brain injury, it is masked in a cloud of anger and sarcasm. I look at that picture and I cry. I mourn the loss of the son that I raised and the future he had planned. I also mourn the loss of the future I planned for myself. That all changed on October 4, 2006, I just had no idea how much.

My son was sixteen years old when he had his car accident. He was supposed to sign paperwork that weekend to join the military and do boot camp the summer between his junior and senior year of high school. My husband and I had just bought a Harley and we had plans of weekend road trips, rides down in the hills and going to flea markets and auctions.

> *"I mourn the loss of the son that I raised and the future he had planned. I also mourn the loss of the future I planned for myself."*

One moment in time was all that it took and suddenly it was gone. Don't get me wrong, I am forever grateful that my son is alive, but there is still a part of me that asks, "Why?" A part of me that feels this is so unfair. The daily struggles are unbelievable. My son is now married and out on his own, so to speak, but it seems like I am called for help with the slightest problem. It seems as though if it can go wrong it does, and he has some of the most unusual luck in the world. I have often told people if I were to write my life story, they would say it was fiction.

After his accident I was given some paperwork about teenagers and TBI's. There were some behaviors that the paperwork said might occur. My son hit every one of them! He started smoking, drinking, we had a couple of run-ins with the law, and drug use. You might think that he saw the paper and used it as an excuse, but he never saw it. Even if he had, his reading comprehension after the accident plummeted so he probably wouldn't understand it. I have learned that our society desperately needs to be educated on brain injuries. I have had countless people tell me what I should do - everything from just walking away to actually having him put in a home. Until you have lived this you don't understand and claiming that you do is somewhat insulting.

The first time my son went to jail I couldn't visit him for over a week because he didn't have the visitation paper filled out. I finally got someone to listen to me and I explained that he probably didn't understand what he was reading. She sent someone back to help him fill it out. I watched him go through a hearing where they knew he had a TBI. I saw him plea to a lesser charge only to call me later asking me what happened because he didn't understand. My son is by no means a bad kid, he is a good kid who made some bad choices.

Through all of this there have been bursts of unexplained anger, temper fits when he can't have it his way and spells of depression. Before the accident my son didn't raise his voice to me and rarely argued. Now, it's almost a daily occurrence. No one, even my husband, knows everything that I deal with concerning my son.

The other day someone told me that I should file guardianship papers. His caseworker and doctors agree with me that isn't needed. He has lost so much that if I take away his ability to sign for himself, it would be devastating to him. I just can't do that to my son.

This past summer was one for the record books. I was having a discussion with my son concerning his behavior and choices when I made the comment that his behavior was slowly killing me. I told him that I couldn't keep doing this. I will never forget the words that came out of his mouth next. He told me that he was tired of being different from everyone else. He said that he missed who he used to be and that he fights daily with himself to not do the things he wants to do to himself but won't. He tells everyone suicide is a permanent solution to a temporary problem and the only thing it does is hurt others and leave a lot of unanswered questions.

At the date of writing this my son is over seventy days clean and sober and is attending a local church. He was very lucky that a deputy in our county took an interest in him and wanted to help him. I will be forever grateful to her. I hope that somehow in the near future our society will have the opportunity to educate themselves on TBI's and be more understanding of the survivors and their families. For now, I will continue to do the best I can for both me and my son. We both deserve it.

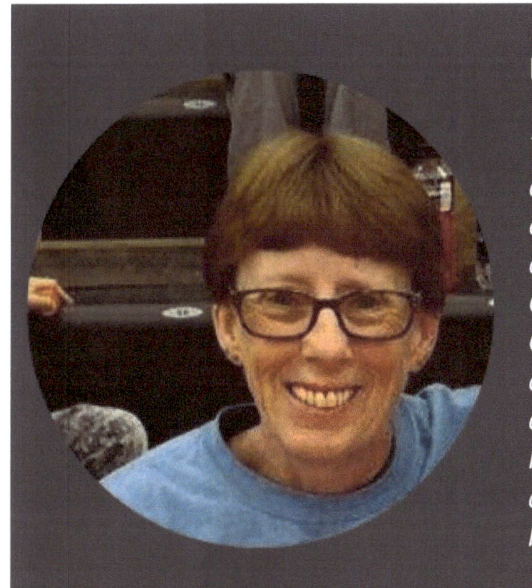

Meet Tracie Massie

Tracie writes… "I live in Darbyville, Ohio and work for our local school as teacher's aide for special needs and IEP students. I am the mother of a TBI survivor. My son's TBI occurred when he pulled out in front of a semi in 2006. He spent three weeks in a coma at Grant Medical Center and spent another six weeks in rehab at Nationwide Children's Hospital. I worked in the healthcare field almost my entire adult life. This was a huge help when it came to caring for my son after the accident, but I really believe his TBI prepared me for the job I have now working with special needs. I have found that it has awakened a passion inside me for helping do all I can for them and be an advocate for them when needed."

"Courage is found in unlikely places."

— J.R.R. Tolkien

Brain Injury Stigmas

By Isaac Peterson

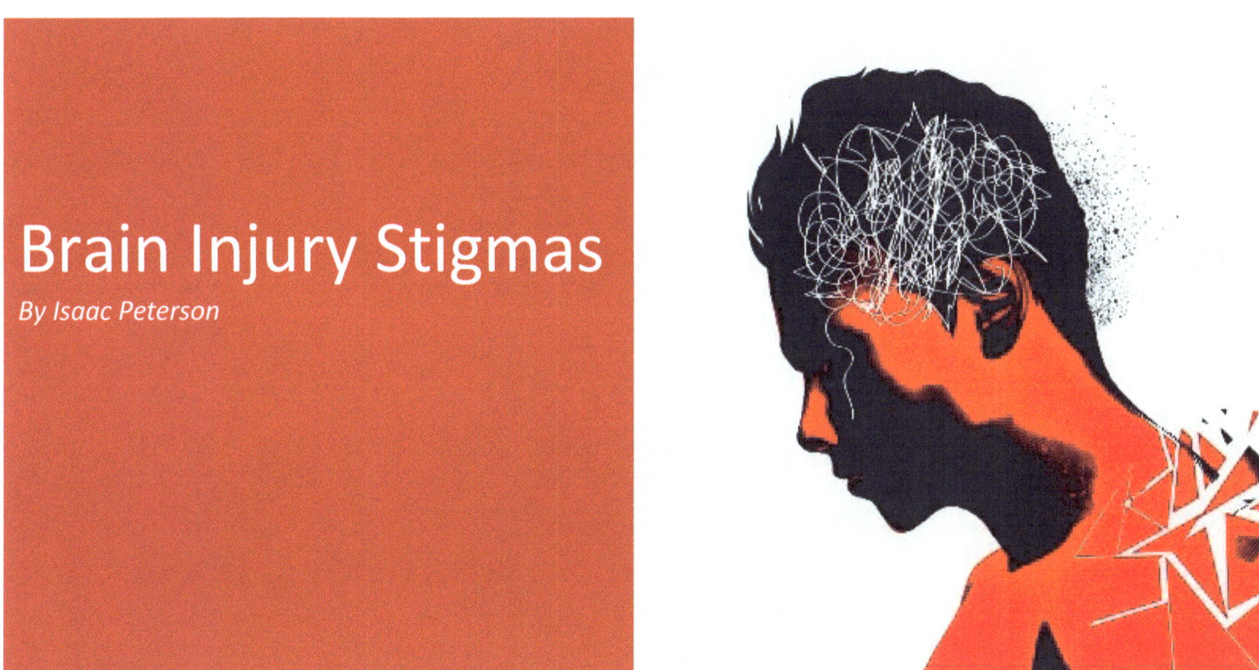

There are some things people say to me that make living with a traumatic brain injury even more of a challenge. Over time, I realized that these were brain injury stigmas.

Stigmas are the preconceived notions people without a traumatic brain injury (TBI) have about us within the brain injury community. At the very minimum, they can be very frustrating, and sometimes discouraging or even hurtful. Many people seem to think traumatic brain injury is the same as brain damage and treat us accordingly. It can lead to people having unrealistic expectations of us. Stigmas can even make them shun us or treat us as less than fully human.

The misunderstanding is theirs, but when they act on those misconceptions, they can make their problem ours. And it happens more than some might realize.

"Stigmas are the preconceived notions people without a traumatic brain injury (TBI) have about us within the brain injury community."

According to recent data from the Centers for Disease Control, 1.7 million people sustain a traumatic brain injury annually. I'm not sure if that figure includes people who already had a TBI and suffered a new one. Some of those people get new injuries by falling and hitting their heads, being in car accidents, or in any number of ways.

The CDC also says that of those 1.7 million people, 275,000 people a year are hospitalized and 52,000 die. There is obviously no way to know how many traumatic brain injuries go unreported. Some people may go a long time between the time of the brain injury and finding out they have one. That's a lot of people in this country with injured brains, and a lot of people with the added burden of having to deal with hurtful stigmas. I have had the misfortune of dealing with many brain injury stigmas. Here is a list of a few stigmas that I have personal experience with. If you are a brain injury survivor, many of these will sound familiar.

Stigma #1: You didn't get hit that hard. You can't have a brain injury.

Oh yes, you can. It really doesn't take that much force to cause your brain to move a bit inside your skull. My TBI–the legacy of a major stroke–is a closed skull TBI. Even I was surprised when I found out that it was considered a brain injury. The bleeding in my brain caused pressure in my skull and gave me a traumatic brain injury.

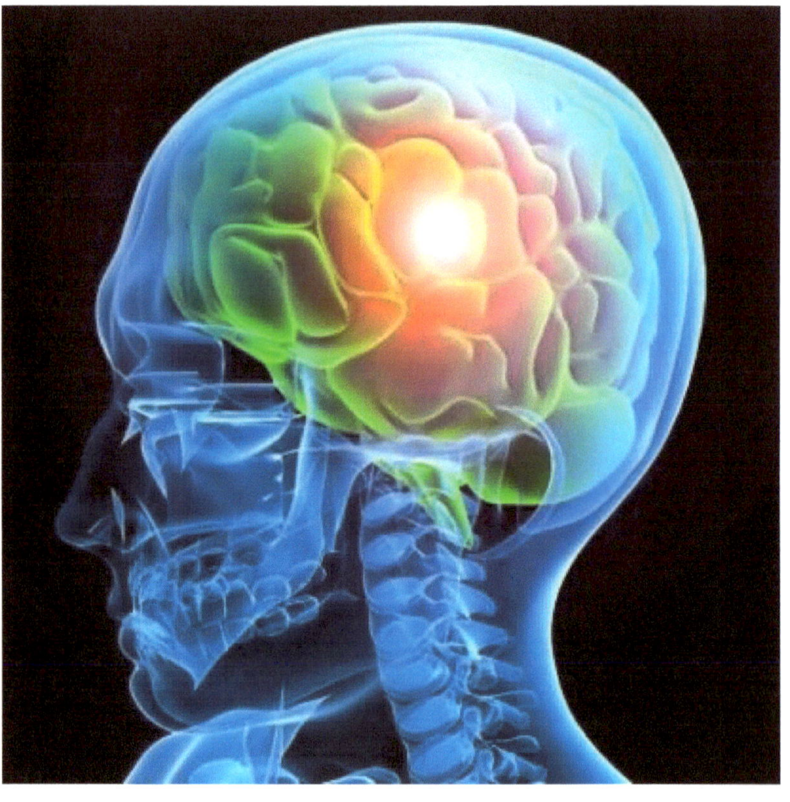

Stigma #2: You didn't get hit in the head, so there's no way you can have a brain injury.

This one is closely related to number one. A direct hit is not necessary to cause a brain injury. As noted above, any event that causes the brain to move inside the skull, like whiplash, may lead to a brain injury. Strokes are also a common form of brain injury.

Stigma #3: You were wearing a helmet. You can't have a brain injury.

Apparently, people seem to forget that even football players who wear helmets every second they're playing can have TBIs. More and more football players are turning up with the form of TBI known as Chronic Traumatic Encephalopathy (CTE), enough that the NFL has been forced to treat it as a major concern. Motorcycle riders who experience crashes can sustain a brain injury even if they show no outward signs of injury.

Stigma #4: You had your brain injury a long time ago. You just want people to feel sorry for you.

No two brain injuries are alike. Since there is no set time for recovery, people take varying amounts of time to recover–if they recover at all. There are people who suffer from TBI for many years. Some suffer for the rest of their lives.

Stigma #5: If you just don't think about it so much, it will go away.

People with a TBI can't help but think about it. They live with a brain injury every minute of every day. There are things that can help people live a bit easier with a brain injury, but even the coping skills they develop are only dealing with the symptoms and not the cause. If a TBI eventually does go away, it will do so in its own time, regardless of whether the sufferer thinks about it or not.

Stigma #6: You can tell if somebody has a brain injury by looking at them.

I have no idea why people think that. As I said about my brain injury, it's of the closed-skull type. Some people think that unless you have a crowbar lodged in your head you can't possibly be injured. They expect all brain-injured people to have some kind of open skull condition. TBI is internal, with no visible outward indicators.

I really can't tell you how to deal with stigmas, though it would be nice if everybody could be educated about traumatic brain injuries, but they aren't. Aside from never leaving the house, it looks like stigmas are simply a part of life for people with TBI. People that perpetuate the stigmas are often people who really do mean well, however they just don't understand what it's like to have a brain injury. All you can realistically do about it is to be patient with them and try calmly to explain. You can use your own experience with brain injury to teach and educate others.

Maybe then they will start to understand.

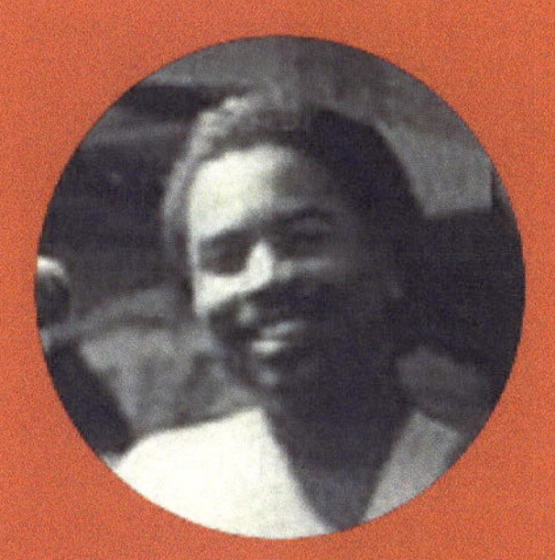

Meet Isaac Peterson

Isaac Peterson grew up on an Air Force base near Cheyenne, Wyoming. After graduating from the University of Wyoming, he embarked on a career as an award-winning investigative journalist and as a semi-professional musician in the Twin Cities, the place he called home on and off for 35 years. He also doesn't mind it at all if someone offers to pick up his restaurant tab.

"It's your life; you don't need someone's permission to live the life you want. Be brave to live from your heart."
— Roy T. Bennett

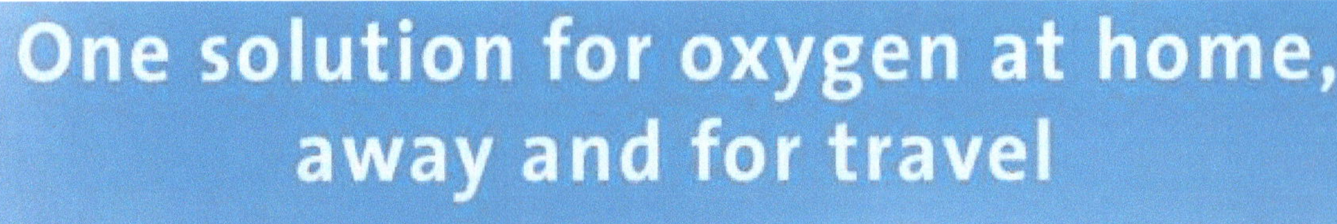

The Caregiver's Caregiver

By Donna O'Donnell Figurski

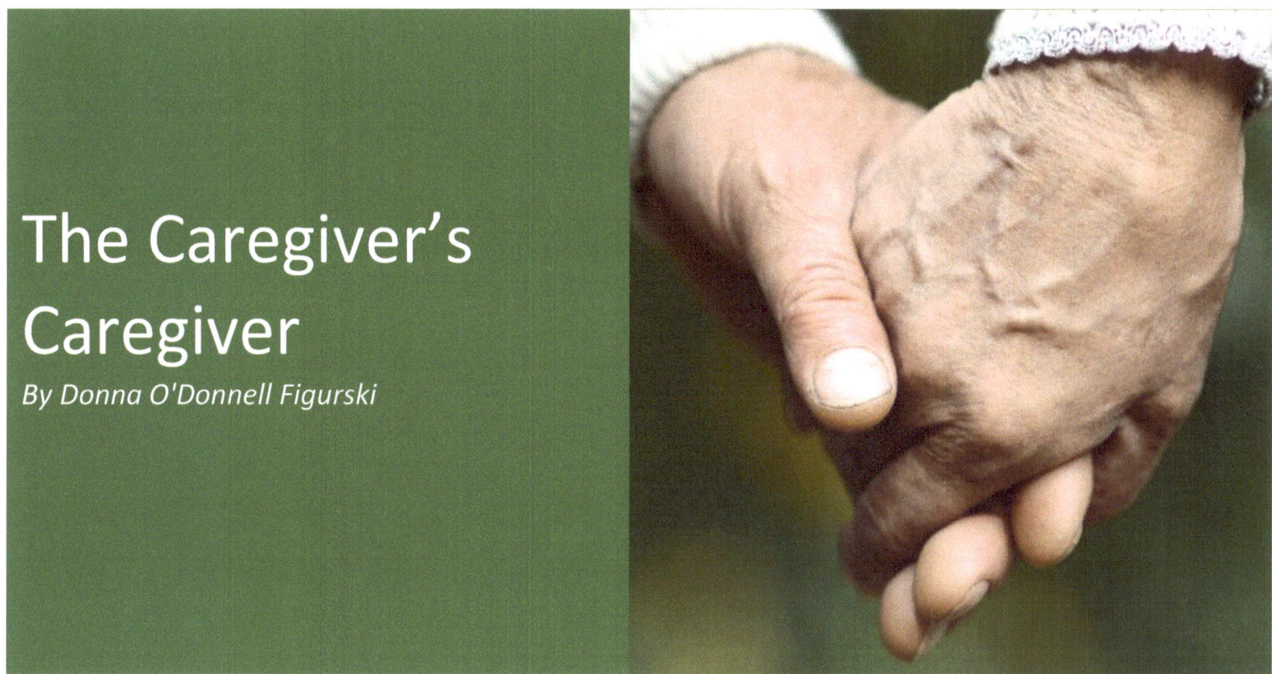

Are you a caregiver? Have you ever been a caregiver? Do you think you ever will be? Stop! Don't answer that. Did you know that according to the U.S. and World Population Clock on the United States Census Bureau website, there are more than 329 million people living in the United States? It is estimated that more than 5 million Americans are living with disabilities relating to brain injury, and many of them need full-time care. Did you know that more than 65 million people are caregivers? With such a high proportion of caregivers, it's not surprising that many of us have worn the caregiver hat at some point in time.

I have, and I still do. I became a forever-caregiver in January 2005, when my husband had a subarachnoid hemorrhage from exercising—from doing thirteen chin-ups. Can you even imagine getting a brain injury from exercising—from trying to keep healthy? Brain injuries happen all the time and sometimes in the strangest ways. It only takes an instant to become a brain-injury survivor, and it takes that same amount of time to become a caregiver.

"A caregiver is a person who voluntarily or, in many cases involuntarily, oversees the health-care and daily needs of another person."

So, what is and who is a caregiver? A caregiver is a person who voluntarily or, in many cases involuntarily, oversees the health-care and daily needs of another person. Often a caregiver is a family member, such as a spouse caring for his or her partner or a son or daughter looking after his or her elderly parents. Sometimes a close friend has taken on the responsibility of managing his or her friend's life. Caregiving often means daily looking in on the care-recipient—perhaps running errands for him or her or preparing a meal. In my case, and in many cases, caregiving is a twenty-four-hour-a-day job every day. Becoming a caregiver can drastically change one's life.

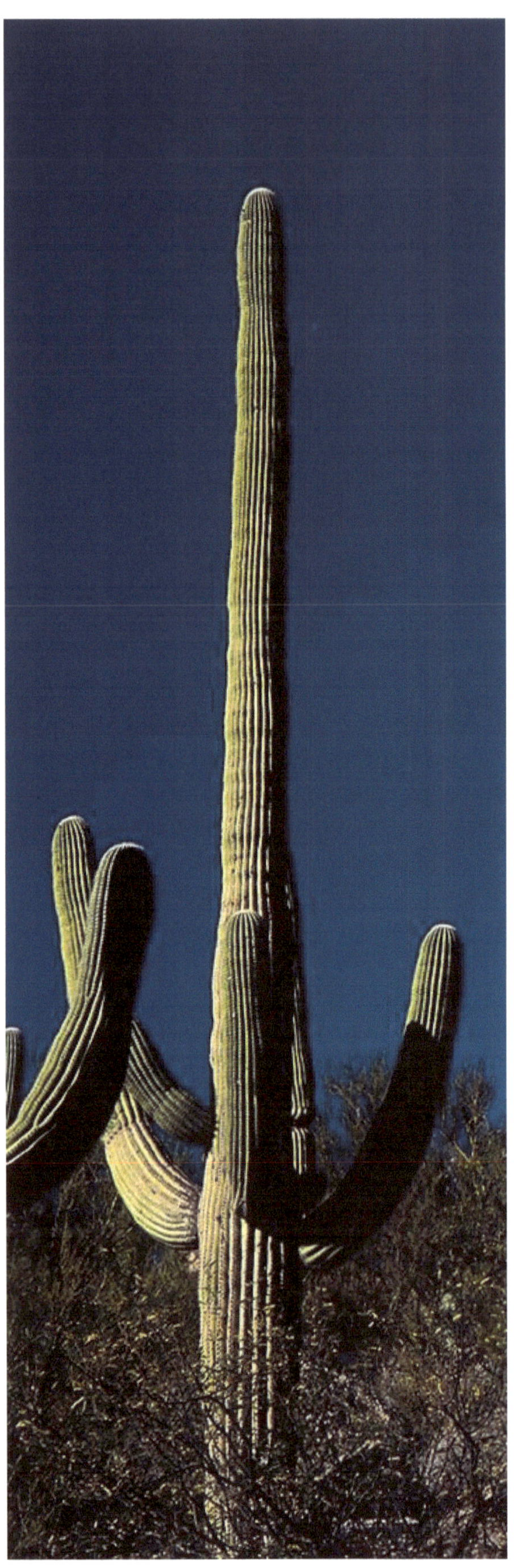

Caregiving usually entails jobs for which most of us have not been trained. Yet, when the need arises, caregivers step forward and learn on the job. I know I did. And, I know that many others do too. Many of us strongly believe it's our responsibility. When our loved one suddenly falls ill, we feel it's up to those of us still standing to help out.

I assure you caregiving is not for the faint of heart. It's a darn hard job! Caregivers must be advocates for their care-recipients. In addition, caregivers may have jobs or careers, or they may have children, who need their love, attention, and guidance. Juggling these major responsibilities can be unnerving and overwhelming for even the most efficient of caregivers. There just aren't enough hours in a day to accomplish everything that must be done by caregivers. Doctors' appointments; rehabilitative therapy sessions; preparing special foods and liquids for breakfast, lunch, and dinner are just some of the extra jobs that compete with children's homework, soccer practices, and bedtime stories.

In the minutes between chores, caregivers need to breathe. Yes, I said "breathe." I know we all do that involuntarily, and we don't often give a thought about that very necessary life-skill. Since caregivers are often operating on autopilot—not thinking of anything but the next chore that needs to be accomplished, they must often be reminded to stop and care for themselves. They have to "breathe"!

If you have ever been a passenger on a plane, you will have heard the attendant say, "In the event of a drop in cabin pressure, put on your oxygen mask first and then help others." Caregivers must etch that thought onto their brains. One cannot effectively help others if one's own resources are depleted, and resources are easily depleted while being a caregiver.

So, what can caregivers do? They need to make their lives a priority. They can recognize that they need quality time in their lives. They can and must eke out time for themselves—even if it's only minutes a day. Caregivers need to do something they enjoy—whether it be reading a chapter of a book, taking a walk in the park, running laps in the gym, watching a ball game, or taking a bubble bath. It doesn't matter. What matters is that caregivers take a break, reset their minds, and focus on something less stressful than the constant care of a loved one.

It's hard for caregivers to follow through on self-care when the responsibilities for their care-recipients are looming, but it's important. Burnout and depression are waiting in the wings to overtake the caregiver's life.

I know. I came close. I worked all day as a first grade teacher, ran errands during my one-hour commute home, and then I prepared meals, doled out pills, and tackled household chores, like doing the laundry, before I completed my planning for the next day's schoolwork.

Fortunately, after five years of this schedule, David was secure enough to remain home by himself for an hour or two, and I volunteered in the theater. That was my release. That was my bubble bath. Working in the theater completely immersed me in a different world. It allowed me to recharge. It refreshed my thinking, and it gave me a respite from all my caregiver-duties for a short time.

Many caregivers need to be reminded to take precious time for themselves. In their busy lives, they often don't remember to stop—to smell the roses or whatever flower they like. So, a little reminder is helpful.

I carry a small, black, polished stone with me at all times. I call it a "Me Time Stone." It can be hidden in a pocket or in my bag. Whenever I see it or feel it, it is a constant reminder that I must take a few minutes for me.

> "It's hard for caregivers to follow through on self-care when the responsibilities for their care-recipients are looming, but it's important."

I also keep Me Time Stones on my bathroom vanity, on my bedside table, and at my computer work areas, so I always have a reminder that I am important too. Caregivers need that reminder, but they don't need a black, polished stone. It can be any stone that he or she finds on the ground. I urge the caregiver to choose a Me Time Stone that resonates with him or her because it will soon become the caregiver's caregiver.

Did you know that just about everyone is, has been, or will be a caregiver at some point in his or her life? That's what former First Lady Rosalyn Carter said … "There are only four kinds of people in the world - those who have been caregivers, those who are caregivers, those who will be caregivers and those who will need caregivers." Which one are you?

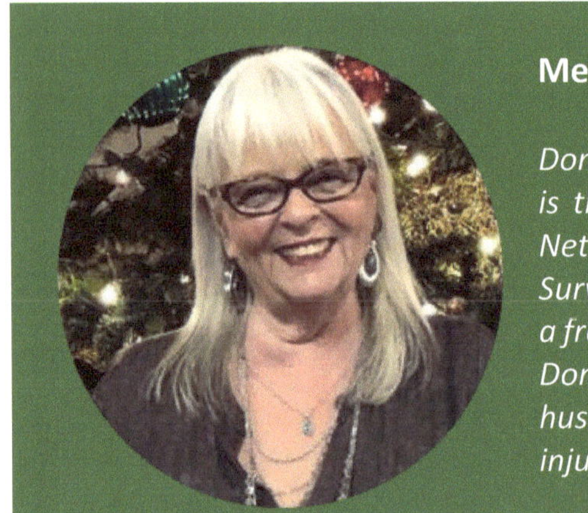

Meet Donna O'Donnell Figurski

Donna is the author of Prisoners without Bars: A Caregiver's Tale. She is the host of "Another Fork in the Road" on the Brain Injury Radio Network and is the creator and writer for her award-winning blog, Surviving Traumatic Brain Injury. As a brain-injury advocate, Donna is a frequent contributor to both print and online journals and magazines. Donna claims her greatest accomplishment is being caregiver to her husband and high school sweetheart, David, who had a traumatic brain injury in 2005. She and David live in the Arizona desert.

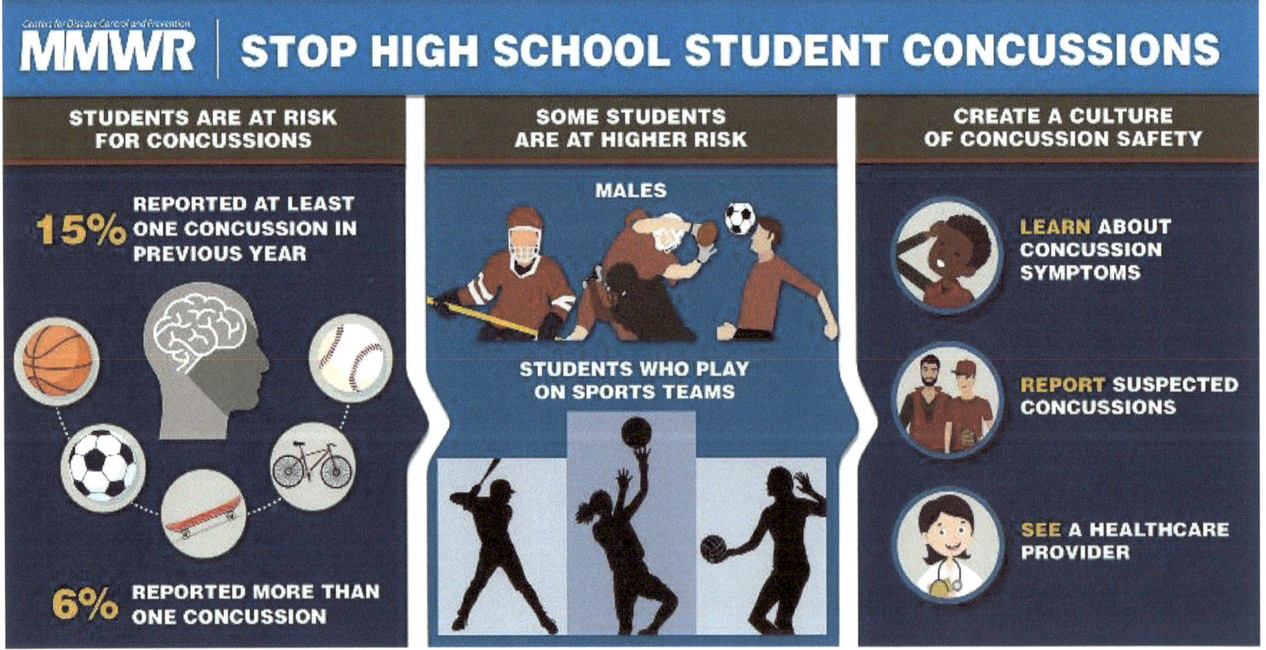

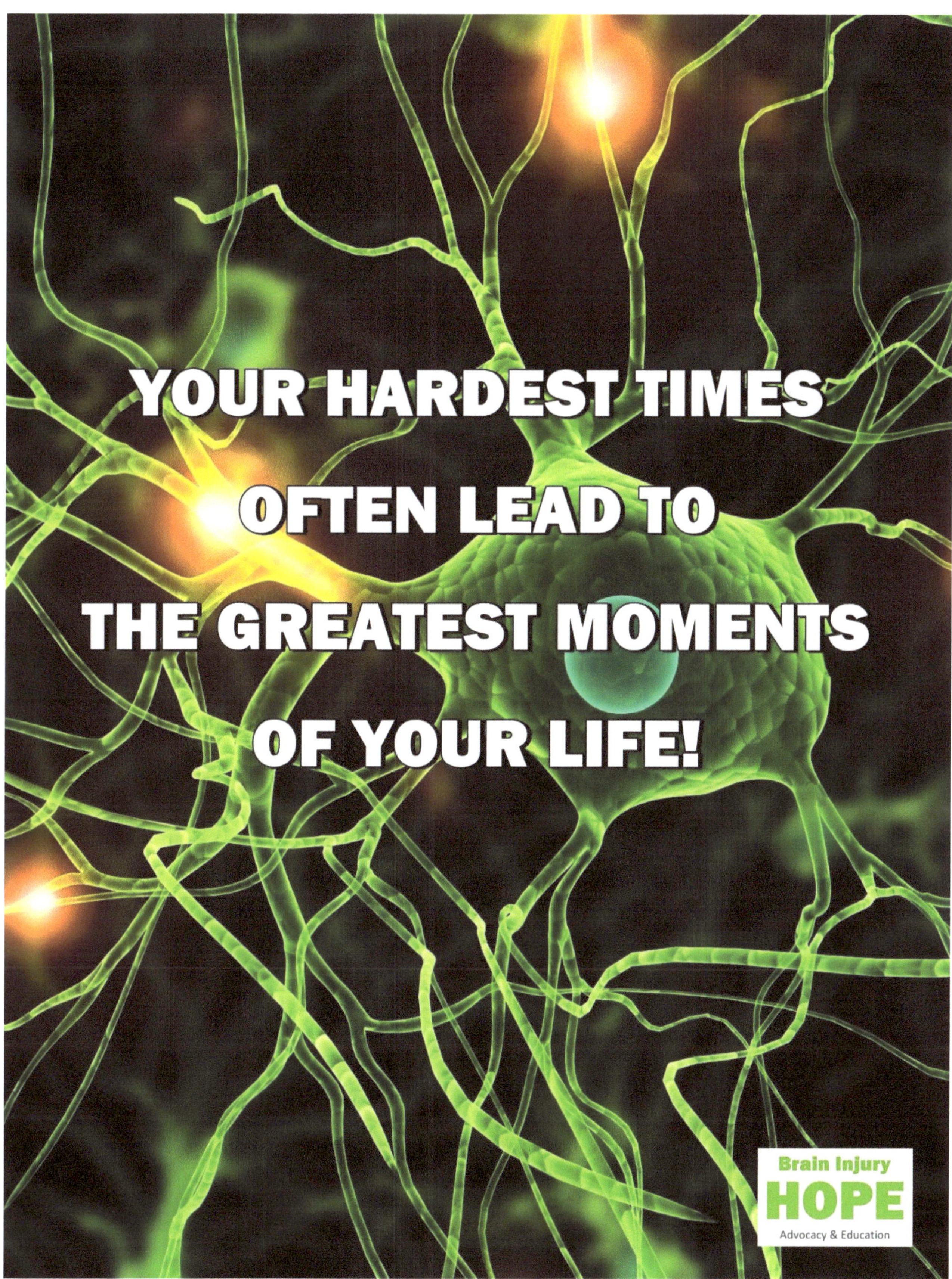

YOUR HARDEST TIMES
OFTEN LEAD TO
THE GREATEST MOMENTS
OF YOUR LIFE!
Brain Injury
HOPE
Advocacy & Education

Shaken

By Susan Hayes

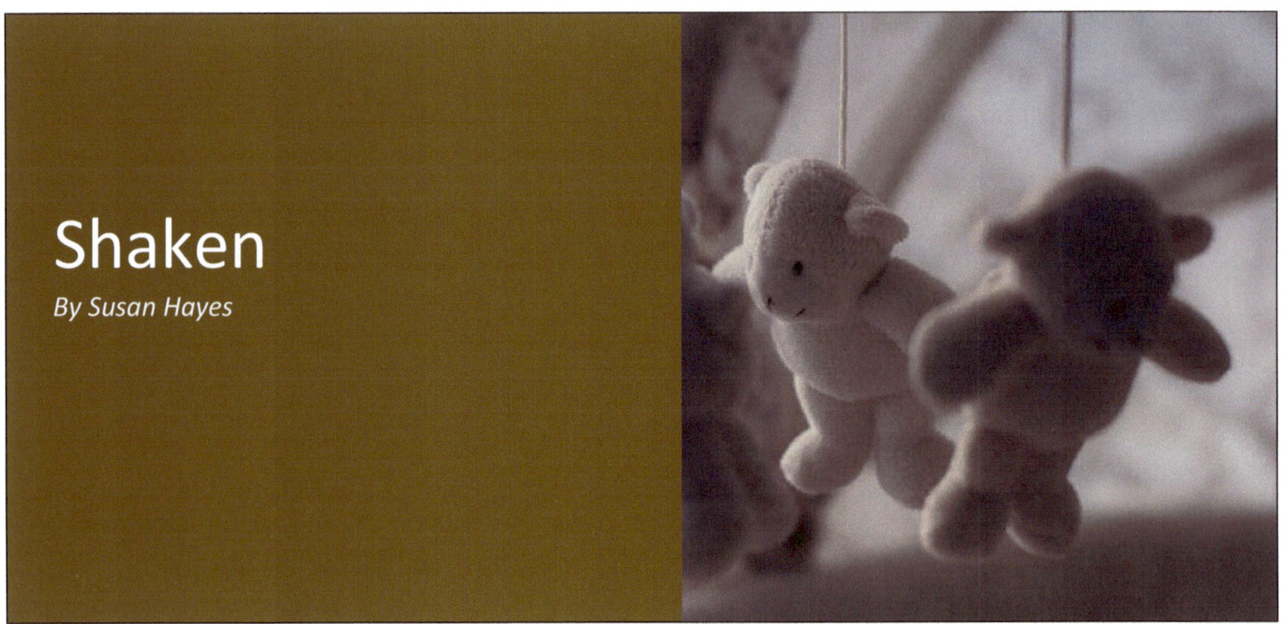

Isaiah was born on October 8, 2007, 6 pounds 4 ounces and 12.5 inches long. Two days later he went home with us as a happy baby. He was meeting or exceeding every milestone that he was supposed to and he was strong. In June of 2008 I was working full-time. June 11th started like every other weekday. Isaiah was dropped off at his babysitter's and his older two siblings went to a daily summer camp. I had just gotten back from my afternoon break when I got a phone call at work. It was the babysitter. She said that Isaiah had fallen out of the crib and was not breathing. I remember telling her I was on my way and running out of my work area. I do not remember telling anyone where I was going.

> *"I recall Isaiah lying lifeless in the babysitter's arms making sounds like a dying animal."*

I called my mom, who I had carpooled with, and told her to come and get me. I had a feeling that I could not stand there and wait, so I started walking. I got several more calls on my cellphone while I walked, and just kept saying that I was on my way. The babysitter sounded more frantic with every call. As I was walking, I was picked up by the babysitter's husband who drove me the rest of the way. I do not know how long it took for me to get from work to their house, but the world stopped the minute I saw Isaiah. I recall Isaiah lying lifeless in the babysitter's arms making sounds like a dying animal. He grunted and pushed against me and he would calm down when I would talk to him and whisper in his ear. I called my mom again and told her we were headed to the emergency room.

The emergency room experience is a blur. When we walked into the emergency room, the intake staff looked at my limp baby in my arms and took us straight back to a room. They asked what happened. I told them that the babysitter said he fell out of the crib. They put him in a neck brace, and they raced him to x-ray and ordered a CT scan. I sat with him on the gurney the whole time. They put an IV in his arm and gave him medication to calm him. They had braces on his arms to prevent movement because of the IV. Isaiah's breathing got shallow so they made me leave the room so that they could intubate him.

The doctors came to me in the adjoining examination room and said Isaiah needed to go to one of the children's hospitals. They asked if we wanted to go to Seattle or Denver. The first thing I thought was, "Why do we need to go somewhere else? Can't we stay here?" Then the next thoughts that entered my head were, "Why are you asking me where I want to go? You are the doctors. You should know where to send him." I finally asked them where they thought we should go. We decided on Denver Children's Hospital. I was then rushed to a waiting ambulance that would take us to the airport to be Life Flighted to Denver.

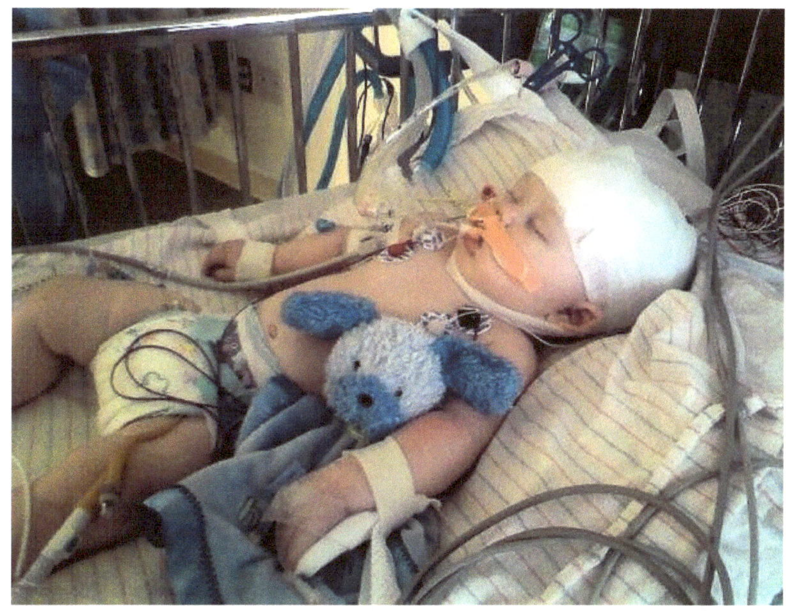

Once we got to the hospital in Denver, it was a blur of noises and sights. In the emergency room at Denver Children's Hospital, I was handed paperwork to complete. I do not remember much about the paperwork, because I was staring at a yellow curtain that was closed to onlookers. I saw doctors and nurses going quickly in and out of that curtained area. Then we were rushed up to the Pediatric Intensive Care Unit (PICU). The lack of noise was a shock compared to the sounds of the emergency room. The only noise was the beeping of machines. I went to sleep in Isaiah's room listening to the beeping of the machines making sure he was still alive. The next morning, the parade of caseworkers and doctors all started asking questions and giving perceptions of what may have happened to Isaiah.

The first time we got any real information was when Isaiah started having seizures. We had been moved to a regular room for about a week after we had gotten to Denver. We stayed in that room for one night before he started seizing. The seizures were causing his vital signs to drop drastically. We were asked to leave the room because the doctors had to intubate him again and drain the fluid that had accumulated on his brain. That is when one of the neurologists told us how serious the injuries were to Isaiah's brain. The neurologist showed us the magnetic resonance imaging (MRI) and explained that 90% of Isaiah's brain was damaged.

Isaiah ended up in the PICU for several more days. A few days later the ophthalmologist came and evaluated Isaiah. We were told the extent of the damage to his eyes. He had bilateral retinal hemorrhaging.

Once Isaiah was in a regular hospital room, things gradually improved. Isaiah had to get a swallow test. This is where they have him drink a substance that can be seen on an x-ray to make sure liquids were not being aspirated (going into the lungs). He was able to drink formula, so they removed the

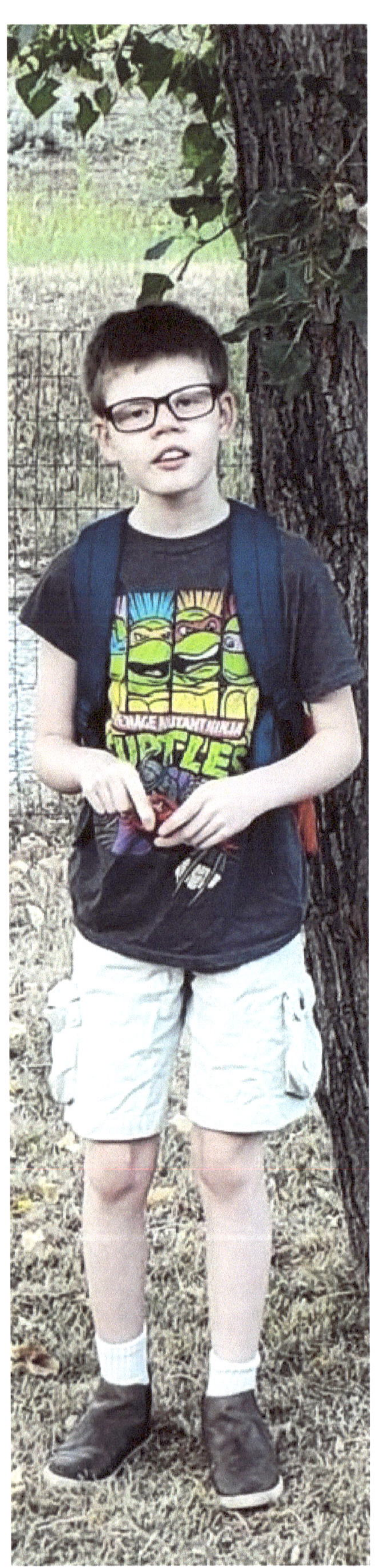

feeding tube. He was prescribed two anti-seizure medications and one antacid to counteract the side effects of one of the medications. After about three-and-a-half weeks in Denver, on June 30, 2008, Isaiah was finally sent home. The doctors predicted that Isaiah would never have a normal life. With the extent of his injuries, doctors did not expect him to survive past his first birthday. The doctors also stated that he would probably never walk or talk.

Today Isaiah is a very active and talkative young man. The road has been an uphill struggle and will continue to be one. Isaiah traveled to Denver ten times in the first five-and-a-half years. He still has regular appointments with specialists. Isaiah has had a total of four eye surgeries to repair the damage in his eyes.

Isaiah was seizure free for almost three years. He started having seizures again in 2012. He has absence seizures or petit mal seizures. Isaiah's seizures have been mapped to the right frontal lobe of his brain. Now he is partially seizure-free with medication. He takes two types of seizure medications twice daily and an ADHD medication and several other medications to counteract the side effects. He still has breakthrough seizures occasionally and the doctors continue to adjust medications to keep his seizures under control so he can have a semi-normal life.

Academically Isaiah is unable to retain information for long periods of time. He learns new things, but if this information is not continually used, he does not retain the skills. He does not have the vocal capacity of a child his age, therefore he struggles to vocalize what he has done throughout the day.

He can vocalize more in regard to his wants. Self-sufficiency is also a struggle for Isaiah. He cannot dress or bathe himself. It is difficult to keep him under control. He has no inhibitions and he is very strong for his age. He does want to try to do things for himself and cannot always succeed.

Since June 11, 2008 I have lived in a hospital room for several weeks with Isaiah hooked to a machine and tubes. I have attended workshops, seminars, and learning weekends to reach out to others in the healing process. I have seen the inside of a courtroom. I have sat in the witness stand. I have been asked a barrage of questions pertaining to how I take care of my children. I have sat in a waiting room worried about my baby. I have travelled several thousand miles. I have read many medical books in an effort to make sense of what my child is enduring. I divorced, but later married an incredible man, David, who supports me and loves our family unconditionally.

I watched the life of a woman I thought I could trust be destroyed by one act. I watched my life change dramatically because of one act. I watched my children's lives be changed because of one act. I see the world through different eyes. I see the way people look at me when my son is having a meltdown because he cannot explain himself or he is tired or overstimulated. I have been told, "He looks so normal." This is not a compliment. He does look like any other child, but he is a special young man that holds my heart.

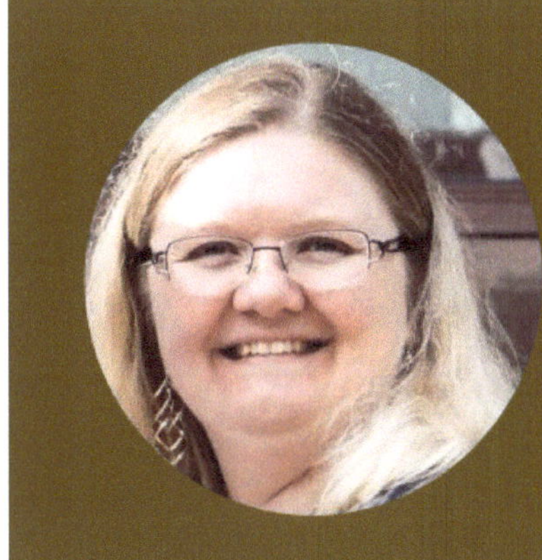

Meet Susan Hayes

Susan writes… "I am almost 40 years old. I am a teacher in a rural school district. I have 3 wonderful children and a terrific husband. We live in central Montana. I hope that by sharing Isaiah's story I can help others know that it is ok to be frustrated, but just to make sure the baby is safe and walk away or ask for help. Shaken Baby Syndrome is real, and it only takes a moment to cause permanent damage."

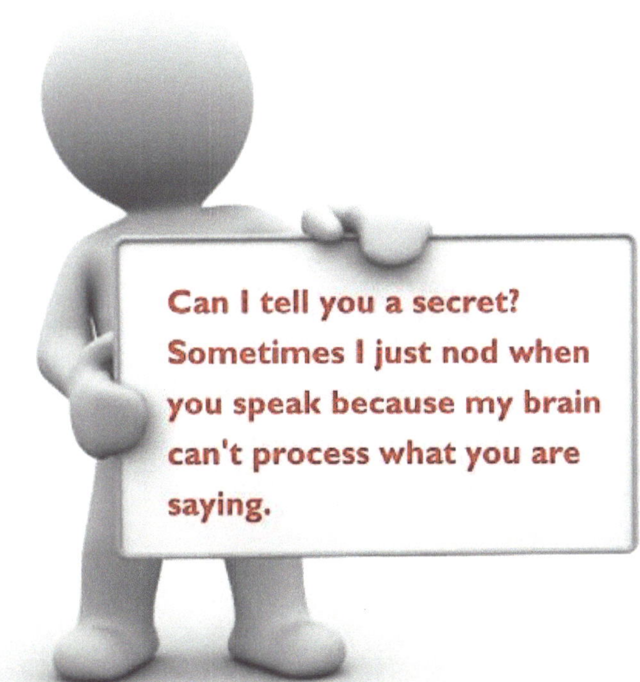

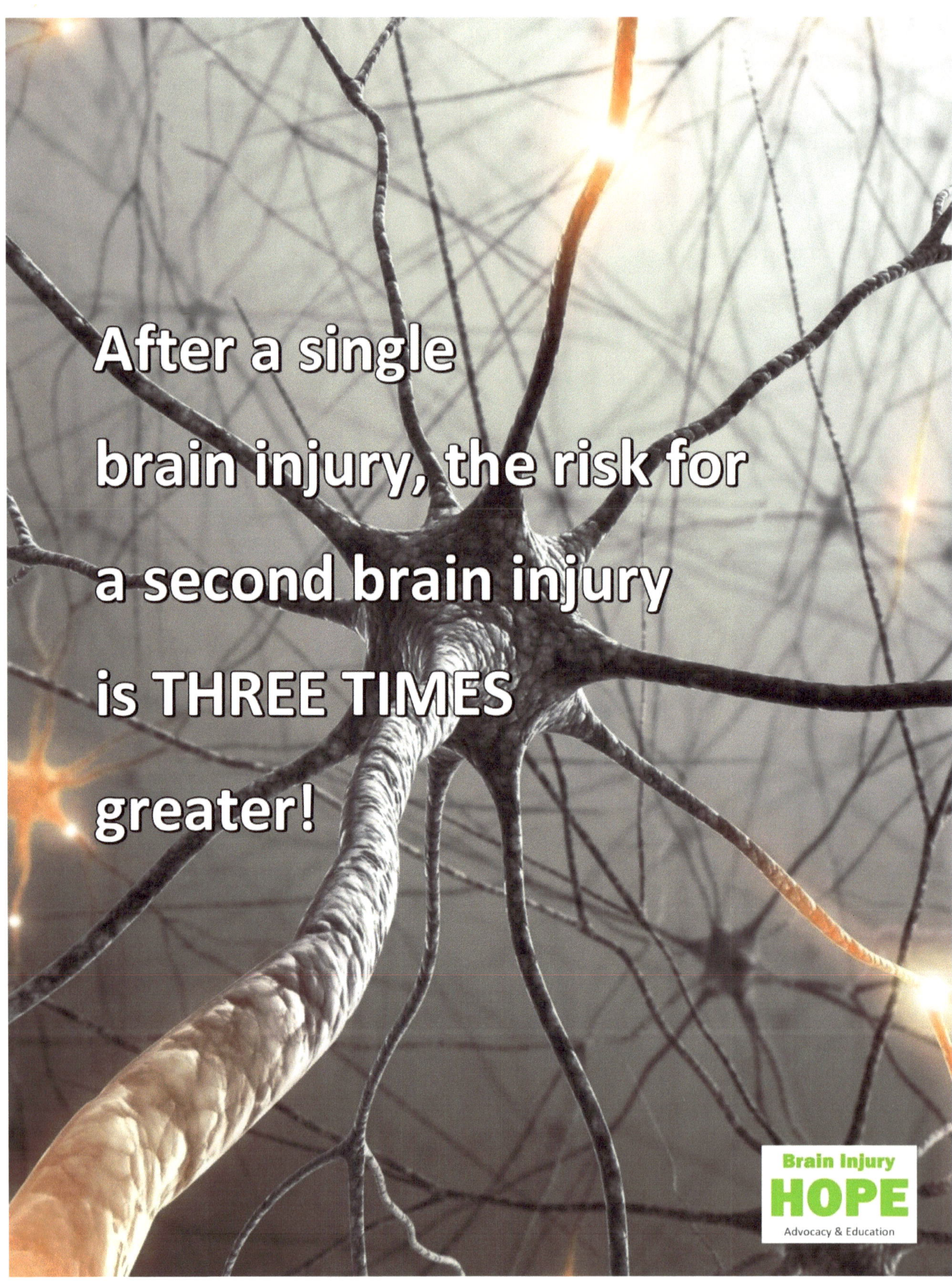
After a single

brain injury, the risk for

a second brain injury

is THREE TIMES

greater!

Brain Injury
HOPE
Advocacy & Education

Finding Hope

By JoAnne Silver Jones

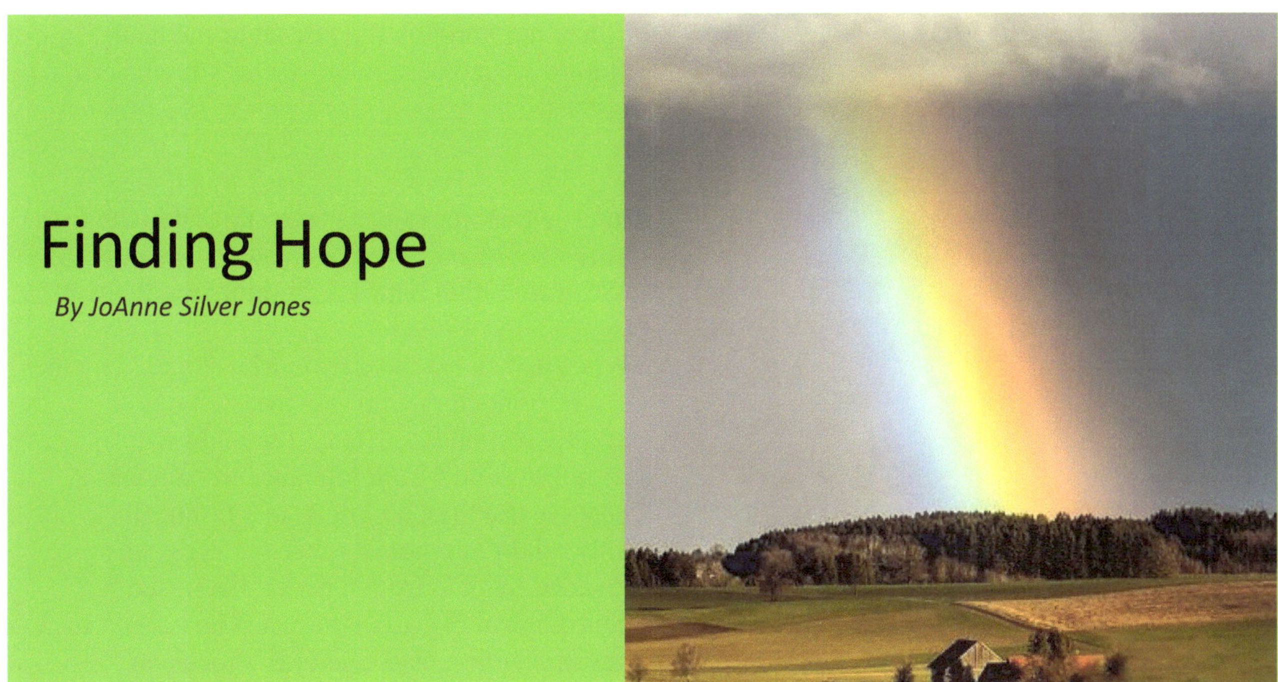

My mother loved to tell the story of when she was six and jumped on an ice delivery truck. "A block of ice fell on me," she'd proclaim, and then laugh and say, "So I just got up and caught the next ice truck that came by!" The moral of this story never changed: get up and get going again. Complaining was the arena of the weak. She was oldest of seven, born to immigrant parents and she learned at an early age to fend for herself, take care of younger siblings and manage, regardless of the circumstances. She passed these lessons to me, through her words and actions.

Our family religion was politics. Beginning in their teen years, both my mother and father became involved in progressive political movements. Critiquing the news of the day was the focus of our dinner conversation. While culturally Jewish, they eschewed religious references and observances of any kind. This message was also passed to me and my brother. Now, I would describe their beliefs with the Hebrew term, *Tikun Olam*, the instruction to Jews to repair the world and to work for justice. I took this instruction to mean that the concerns of the world were more important than my own worries.

"These lessons were imbedded in me when I was attacked by a stranger, just before the inauguration of President Obama. Soundlessly, he beat me with a hammer and left me bleeding in a cold alley, my skull cracked and both hands fractured."

Keep going, regardless. Repair social problems. Avoid organized religion.

These lessons were imbedded in me when I was attacked by a stranger, just before the inauguration of President Obama. Soundlessly, he beat me with a hammer and left me bleeding in a cold alley, my skull cracked and both hands fractured.

With the help of wonderful health professionals and a sea of family and friends, I began the long trek of healing, through the thicket of medical, emotional and cultural obstacles strewn across my path.

As soon as possible, I got back up on the ice truck. I took more steps than suggested the first time I could get out of bed and walk. I put up with pain rather than ask for more medication.

When asked, "How are you Mrs. Jones?" by the scores of doctors who saw me each day, I usually responded, "fine." I thought demonstrating a high tolerance to pain was a positive trait, not an impediment to healing. My father didn't complain when his body was invaded by pain from a never-diagnosed neurological disease. And when he was hit by a bus in San Francisco, he didn't focus on himself. He exercised Tikum Olam when learning that the accident could have been avoided by the addition of a small, extra mirror on the bus's passenger side mirror. He fought for justice and won. All buses now have this mirror. His own suffering was subsumed by larger issues.

It never occurred to me to ask why my head throbbed all the time or why I couldn't look up without pain or why I was always enveloped by relentless fatigue. I constantly and silently worried about what might happen next inside my brain and thought that if I just knew more, I could control more. During the months and early years of recovery, I was often depressed, an emotion my mother didn't believe in. I was reluctant to leave my house. I was seldom excited, but I forged on with exercise and trying to complete daily tasks.

My strategies for dealing with all of the sequelae from the assault were concrete. Do this. Learn that. Practice. Try. Read. My body was healing, but my spirit was somnolent.

Then, for reasons I can't articulate, I started to write, haphazardly at first. As I wrote I began to think of family stories, like the ice truck story, and began to see the connection between the stories and my responses to what had happened to me. Being just fine. Not asking for help. Treating pain as if it were a secret I couldn't let out. Managing, Gritting through. These responses were not only counter-productive to recovery, they weren't true. I wasn't fine. I did have pain. I was depressed.

Recovery meant sorting through the messages of my childhood and prying them loose from where they had resided for so many years. As with other parts of telling my story, decoupling directives from the parents I dearly loved and erecting my own guideposts was a difficult task. I knew it was necessary in order to have agency over my recovery.

I needed more than physical recuperation. I needed something to bolster my heart.

There is no particular moment or event or person I can point to and say, "That's when a change happened." As I wrote, and during the spaces between putting words on paper, I recalled the stories from conversations with different people, or notes in get well cards. I let the love from others soak into me. I remember stories strangers told me about their own process of recovery and began to search for not what was practical, but what could sustain me; what could give me inner strength.

While still enmeshed in the process of writing, and looking for sources of internal direction, I met a flight attendant on a cross country fight. When she opened the overhead compartment near me, a suitcase fell on my head.

I shrieked and my story came pouring out, along with tears. She brought me an icepack and a cup of tea. Shortly after, I went into the galley where we talked effortlessly and eagerly for the reminder of the flight.

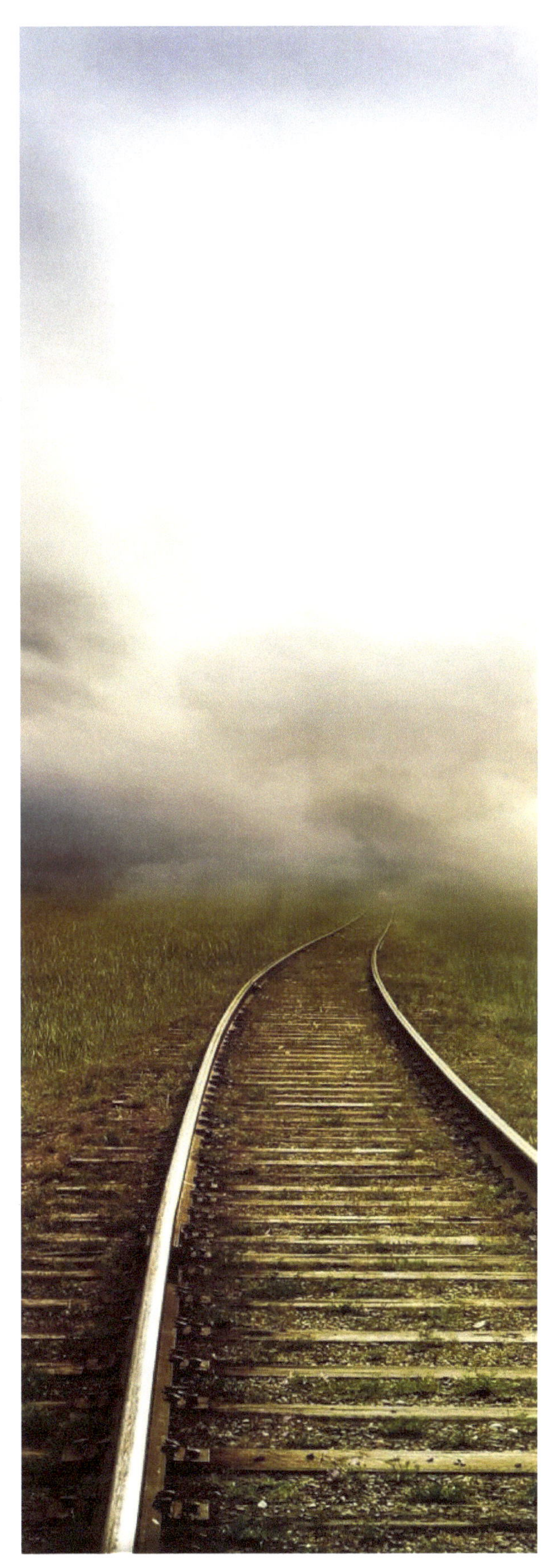

I told her about what happened to me, she told me about her life experiences. I felt alive and hopeful, as our sisterhood at 35,000 ft. developed.

 When I returned to my seat she said, "I'm glad you're here."

I said in response, "So am I."

Her words stayed with me and I remembered a line from a May Sarton poem, "Crazy human with hope." Once the word hope entered my mind, I knew it was the missing piece of my recovery. Maybe it was crazy to be guided by something ineffable. But I knew, with certainty, that hope was the light that would guide me forward. The word for hope in Hebrew is *"Tikvah,"* meaning to gather into strength. Tikvah is not something out of reach, though it does imply waiting patiently amidst the greys of uncertainly, knowing that clarity will emerge in the full technicolor of life.

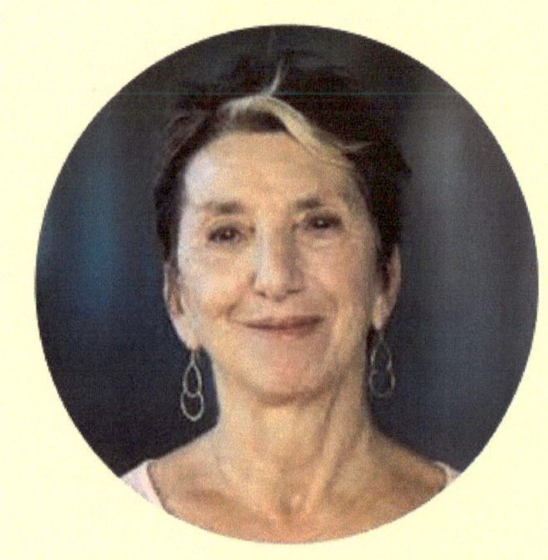

Meet JoAnne Jones

JoAnne was senselessly attacked by a stranger with a hammer to the head. After this sudden assault left JoAnne, a professor and Associate Dean for 25 years in Massachusetts, with severe traumatic brain injury (TBI), fractured hands, and PTSD, she learned—with the help of a community that gave her the foundations of hope—to live with TBI in a society bursting with violence. Her teaching and research focused primarily on social justice issues and her book Headstrong: Surviving a Traumatic Brain Injury published in November 2019.

Living With Hope

By Patrick Brigham

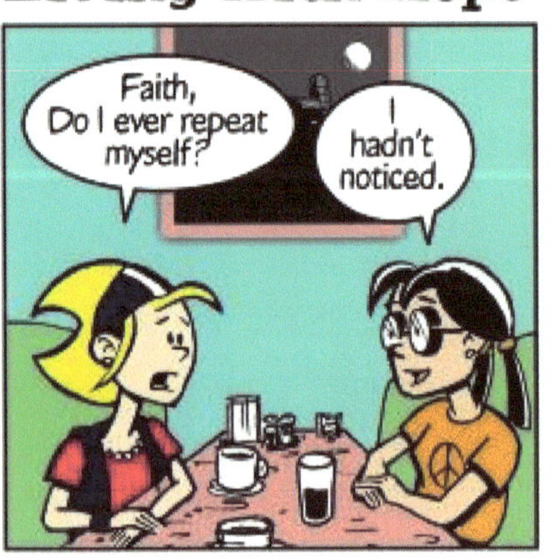

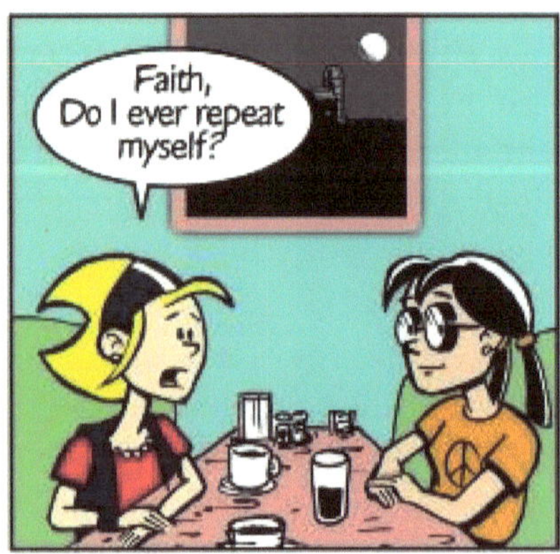

One of the Lucky Ones

By Sandra Bastinelli

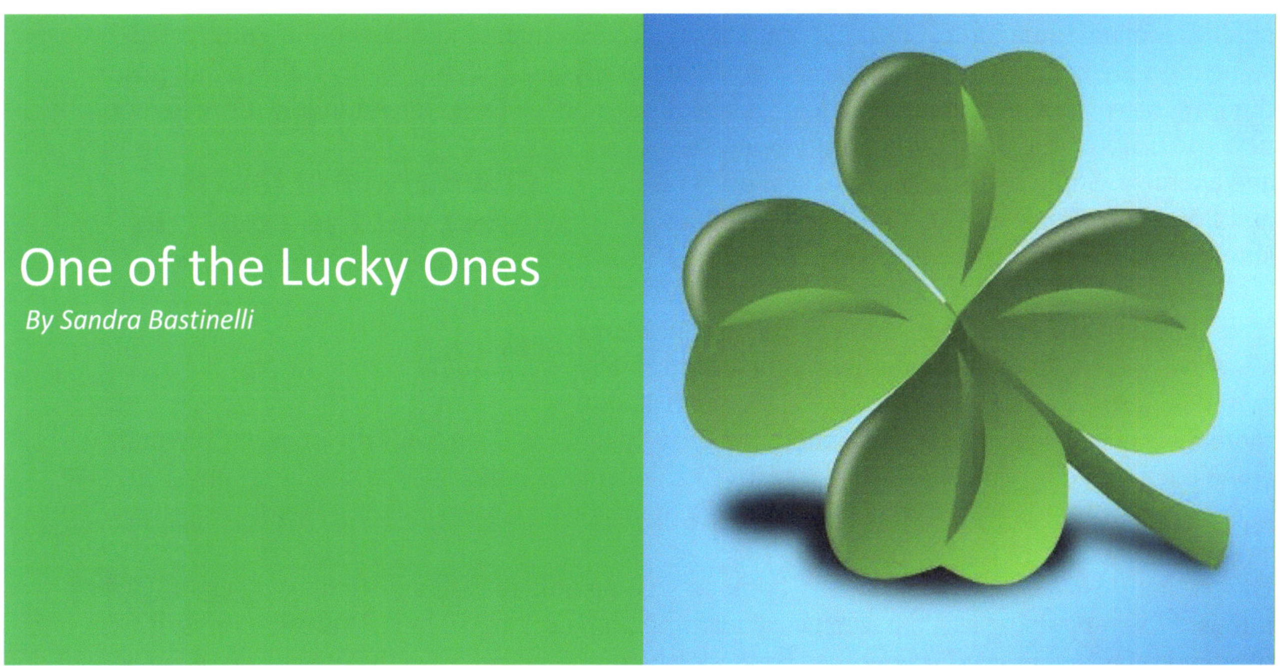

I should know a lot about the brain since healthcare has been my life. I have worked in hospitals and other health care organizations for about fifty years. However, forty years ago Traumatic Brain Injury (TBI) had no meaning. All I knew about brain injury was that a stroke was a brain injury. I worked in a highly competitive, stressful government job for fifteen years.

My snow skiing vacations were my life. I always wanted to learn how to ski and after many years I was considered to be a good skier. In January of 2014, I fell in love with what is considered the highest ski slope in the northeast. I skied this trail several times. This was unusual because I always wanted to try something new. On my sixth time down, my husband saw that I inadvertently skied into an ungroomed area and was careening down the mountain on my face. My skis were somewhere, but thankfully I always wore a ski helmet.

As my husband started to give me CPR, the ski safety staff arrived. An ambulance was called and one of the paramedics stated that I needed to be air lifted to the nearest hospital as traveling by ambulance would take an hour and I was not expected to live that long. I have no memory of any of this or much of the next year, thankfully, speaking as a nurse. After being in a coma for several weeks, I woke up and recognized my husband.

I wasn't able to swallow for another month, so I was fed with a feeding tube. My husband tells me that I had to learn how to walk, talk and eat. I was essentially a baby again. I had over a year of speech therapy. The occupational and physical therapy went on for several months. Every year I understand more and am aware more of life. I still have balance issues and get dizzy easily, but that also has improved immensely with functional neurology care.

I know I am one of the lucky ones. First, I was given a second chance at life. Second, I am now able to do anything I want within reason. Third, I have forgiven everyone who did not believe my life was important and chose not to stay in touch. Fourth, I am able to teach others what they should know about traumatic brain injury. Fifth, I regained my driver's license and lastly, I am motivated, though some days are better than others. I could go on about my outlook, but I truly believe that positive thinking of yourself and your "situation" is absolutely the best way to continue your recovery. My new life is about traumatic brain injury facts, nutrition and exercise. Some of us certainly have a difficult life, and I would be lying if I was to tell you that these last six years have been a piece of cake.

> **"I am grateful that my 'work until you can't do anymore' mentality has come back to my new brain."**

You definitely get out of life what you put into it. I have a list everyday with duties, errands, etc. that need to be completed. More times than not, I have accomplished more than I have scheduled. I am grateful that my "work until you can't do anymore" mentality has come back to me. I realize now that cognitive exhaustion is nothing even similar to physical exhaustion. If I push myself too much, my body just stops working.

By making mistakes, falling inside my home, not being able to read a difficult recipe, and other things, I learn by doing so I am constantly learning about my new brain. I surround myself with people who have my similar beliefs to keep me positive. I realize now that negativity is quite a bit more difficult to deal with when your brain has been injured. Negativity takes all of my energy and my sense of well-being. I have chosen to be cognitively positive. I believe that things happen for a reason and some things take time. Whenever something does not happen the way I expected or wanted, I believe that the outcome was better than I could ever imagine.

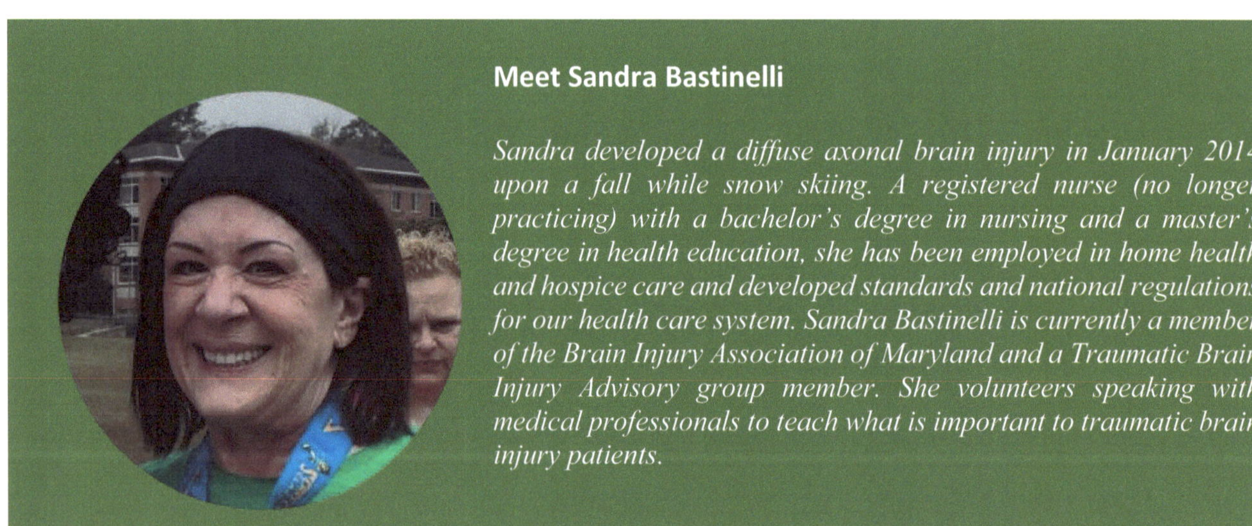

Meet Sandra Bastinelli

Sandra developed a diffuse axonal brain injury in January 2014 upon a fall while snow skiing. A registered nurse (no longer practicing) with a bachelor's degree in nursing and a master's degree in health education, she has been employed in home health and hospice care and developed standards and national regulations for our health care system. Sandra Bastinelli is currently a member of the Brain Injury Association of Maryland and a Traumatic Brain Injury Advisory group member. She volunteers speaking with medical professionals to teach what is important to traumatic brain injury patients.

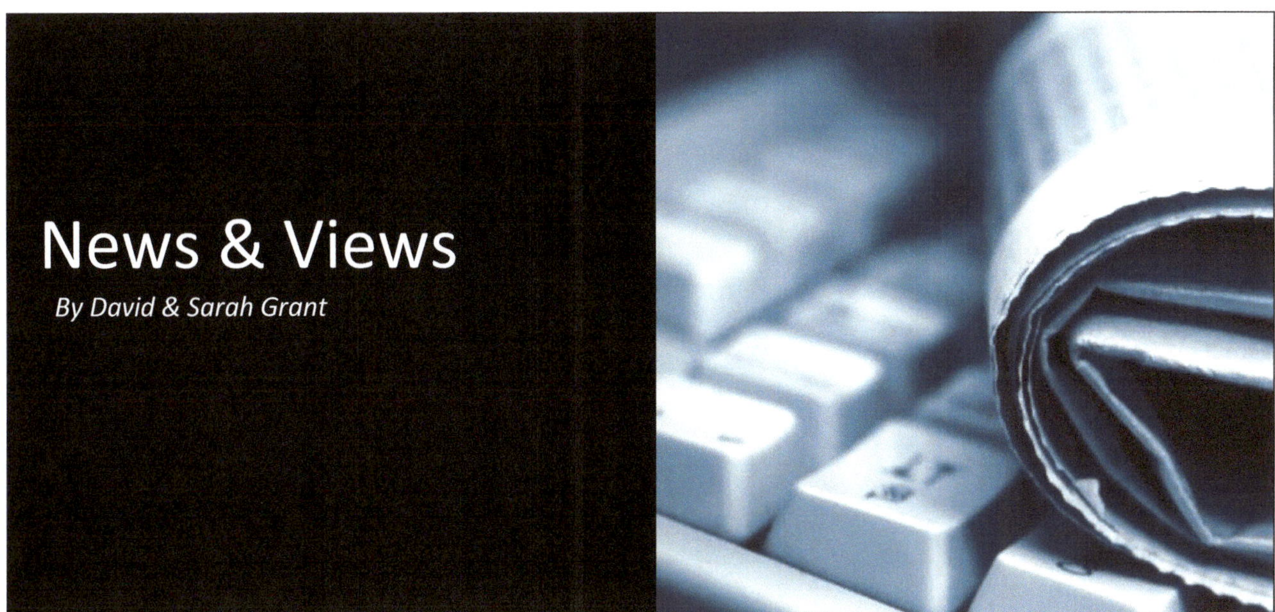

News & Views

By David & Sarah Grant

There is a moment during the production of most every issue of HOPE Magazine that causes both of our hearts to sink. While there is very much the need to let others know, through the sharing of stories, that a meaningful life can be attained after brain injury, it is in the details of the stories themselves that heartbreak comes.

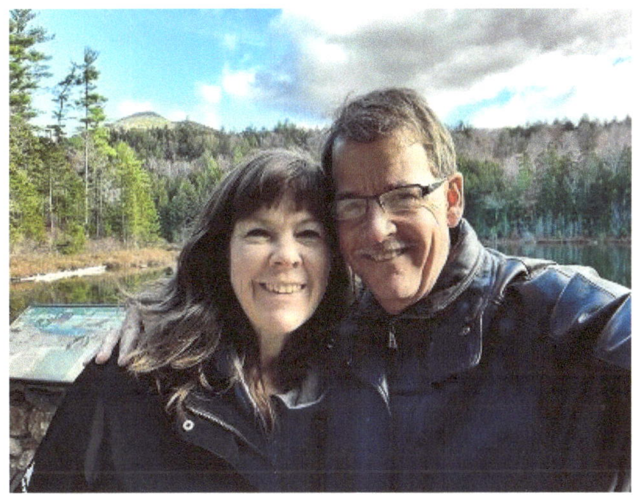

Most every issue that we have produced has at least one "move us to tears" story, courageously shared by a contributor, with the quiet hope that it may help someone else who is struggling.

In this issue, *Shaken* by Susan Hayes was that story.

The very thought of another human being who has acted in such an egregious manner with enough force to cause lifelong injury is difficult enough to fathom. To see that level of violence used in what is essentially an assault on a young baby is nothing short of heartbreaking.

But over the years, we've published other stories that have moved us to tears. There have been countless contributors who have been in motor vehicle accidents. We've shared courageous stories of victims of unwarranted assaults. Domestic abuse has been a recurring theme. Whether by accident, or by the hands of another, brain injury can and does happen every day.

Over the years we have tried to focus on the positives – outcomes that exceed expectations, fellow members of humanity who show stunning kindness, and of course, the quiet connections that happen when one brain injury survivor tries to lift another survivor up – either by words or actions.

To play a small role in facilitating those connections is something that we are profoundly grateful for.

> *~ David & Sarah*